Keto Diet Snack Recipes for Women Over 50

Simple and Tasty Recipes to Burn Fat and Stay Healthy for your Moments of Relax

Rose Pope

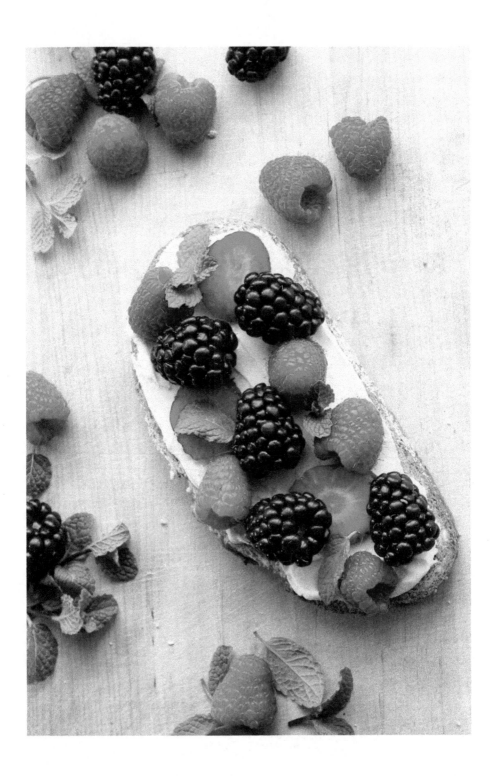

sources. Please consult a licensed professional before attempting any techniques outlined in this book.

By reading this document, the reader agrees that under no circumstances is the author responsible for any losses, direct or indirect, which are incurred as a result of the use of information contained within this document, including, but not limited to, — errors, omissions, or inaccuracies.

Table of Contents

50 Essential Snack Recipes

1   Keto Cucumber Salad

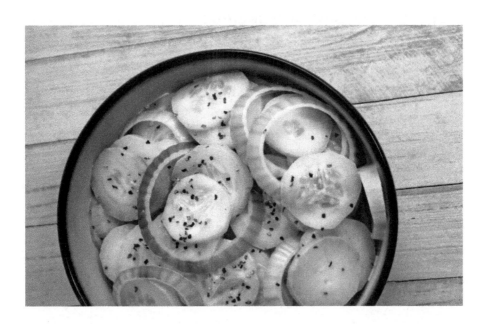

Servings: 4 | **Time:** 3 hrs 15 mins | **Difficulty**: Easy

Nutrients per serving: Calories: 49 kcal | Fat: 3.2g | Carbohydrates: 3.3g | Protein: 1.2g | Fiber: 0.7g

Ingredients

5 Tbsp Full-fat sour cream

2 tsp Fresh dill, minced

1 Large Cucumber, thinly sliced

1 1/2 Tbsp White vinegar

1 1/4 tsp Monkfruit Sweetener (you can use regular sugar too)

1/4 tsp Sea salt, or to taste

1/8-1/4 tsp Black pepper, to taste

1/4 of a Large Onion, sliced thinly

Method

1.   In a big dish, blend all the ingredients until the cucumber is well combined.

2.   Bring the cucumber & onions into the mixture and stir.

3.   To produce flavors, cover, and refrigerate for about 3 hours.

2   Baked Zucchini Fritters

Servings: 16 | **Time:** 45 mins | **Difficulty**: Easy

Nutrients per serving: Calories: 222 kcal | Fat: 21.8g | Carbohydrates: 6.9g | Protein: 3.8g | Fiber: 2.8g

Ingredients

The Fritters:

1 cup Almond flour (100g)

1 Egg white

2 Tbsp of Olive oil, divided

2 tsp Coconut flour

2/3 cup diced Onion

20 Twists Real Salt Organic Garlic Pepper

3 Cups Grated zucchini, packed (2 large zucchinis)

20 Twists Organic Lemon

Pepper

3/4 - 1 tsp Real Salt Sea Salt

6 Tbsp Parsley, minced Olive oil spray

For The Dip:

Real Salt Sea Salt, to taste

5 tsp Fresh lemon juice

4 Twists Real Salt Lemon Pepper

4 tsp Fresh dill, chopped and tightly packed

1/2 Cup Paleo-friendly Mayo

Method

1.   Heat the oven to 400 °F. Line a parchment paper baking sheet. If you have one, use a dark-colored baking sheet as it helps crisp them

2.   Place grated zucchini in the kitchen towel and apply as much moisture as possible to the loop. Put some muscle in it to keep the patties from becoming soggy. In a wide dish, add it.

3.   In a wide skillet, heat 2 tsp of oil over medium heat and set aside the remainder for later. Cook the onion and add it to the zucchini until it's smooth and golden brown.

4.   Add up all the Lemon pepper, parsley, salt, garlic pepper, coconut flour, and almond flour. Stir before it's blended properly. Add the white egg and cook until the zucchini is coated.

5.   Drop 16 meager 1/4 cup balls on the baking sheet - or around 3 Tbsp. Push flat out (approximately 1/4 of an inch) and coat the tops with a spray of olive oil. (You would need to cook in two separate batches)

6.   Bake for about 25-30 minutes, until the sides are golden brown as well as the top becomes slightly crispy. Then, change your oven to broil HIGH and broil for around 2-3 minutes until crisp. Look carefully at how they can burn quickly.

7.   . Mix with all the dip ingredients and DEVOUR with fritters.

3   Keto Paleo Baked Chicken Nuggets In The Air Fryer

Servings: 4 | **Time**: 25 mins | **Difficulty:** Easy

Nutrients per serving: Calories: 286kcal | Fat: 11.6g | Carbohydrates: 10.3g | Protein: 29.9g | Fiber: 5g

Ingredients

Pinch sea salt

A cooking spray of choice

6 Tbsp Toasted sesame seeds

4 Egg whites

1/4 Cup Coconut flour

1/2 tsp ground ginger

1 tsp Sesame oil

1 Lb Free-range boneless, skinless chicken breast

4 tsp coconut aminos (or GF soy sauce)

2 tsp Rice vinegar

2 Tbsp Natural creamy almond butter

1/2 tsp Monkfruit

1/2 tsp ground ginger

1 tsp Sriracha, or to taste

1 Tbsp Water

Method

1.   Preheat the air-freezer for 10 minutes to 400 °F.

2.   Cut a chicken into the nuggets (approximately 1-inch pieces), dry them, and put them in a bowl as the air fryer heats. Toss once covered with the salt and sesame oil.

3.   In a wide Ziploc container, put the coconut flour and the ground ginger and shake to mix. Add a chicken and shake until the chicken is sealed.

4.   Put the egg whites in a wide cup, add the chicken nuggets, and toss them until they are entirely well covered in the egg.

5.   In a large Ziploc bag, put the sesame seeds. Shake the chicken off some extra egg and apply the nuggets to the bag and shake until coated well.

6.   A mesh air fryer basket is generously coated with cooking oil. Put the nuggets in the basket; make sure that they are not crowded or crispy. Spray with the touch of cooking oil.

7.   For 6 minutes, cook. For cooking oil, turn each nugget and spray it. Then cook an extra 5-6 minutes until the interior is no longer pink, with a crispy exterior.

8.   While the nuggets are cooking, in a medium bowl, whisk together all sauce ingredients until smooth. DEVOUR nuggets and serve.

4   Keto Garlic Parmesan Zucchini Fries

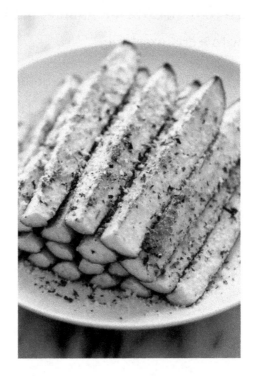

Servings: 6 | **Time**: 40 mins | **Difficulty:** Easy

Nutrients per serving: Calories: 44 kcal | Carbohydrates: 5g | Protein: 3g | Fiber: 1g

Ingredients

4 zucchinis, tops, and bottoms cut off

1 tbsp garlic powder

1/4 cup parmesan cheese, fresh shredded

1/4 tsp salt

1/4 tsp pepper

Method

1.   Preheat the oven to 375 °F.

2.   Halve the zucchini into slices, widthwise.

3.   Again, slice in two, lengthwise.

4.   Slice the halves into four, making long, slender types of fry. If you have a giant zucchini, continue slicing until long, thin strips are available.

5.   Pat with paper towels to rinse.

6.   Toss the garlic powder, salt, parmesan, and pepper in a big bowl over the fries.

7.   Place your fries on a baking sheet with parchment paper. Space out, so the fries don't hit.

8.   Reduce the oven heat to 350.

9.   Based on the size of the fries, bake until crunchy and brown around 20-35 minutes.

10.   If browning fries are too fast, reduce the heat to 300 °F. increase the cooking time.

5 Keto Coleslaw

Servings: 6 | **Time**: 10 mins | **Difficulty**: Easy

Nutrients per serving: Calories: 262 kcal | Fat: 27.42g | Carbohydrates: 2.78g | Protein: 0.56g | Fiber: 1.1g

Ingredients

1 cup mayonnaise

1 tsp toasted sesame oil

1/4 cup sugar-free powdered sugar

10 oz Bag Angel Hair Coleslaw Dressing

3 tbsp white vinegar

Method

1.   Mix the dressing. Taste to change the tastes.

2.   Apply the angel hair slaw to 3/4 of a dressing and turn. Add more if required. Better if consumed within the next few hours.

3.   To Make Ahead: Blend, cover, and then refrigerate dressing for up to 2 days. Only before eating, dress the cabbage.

6 Keto Chorizo Stuffed-Mushrooms with Cheese

Servings: 6 | **Time:** 40 mins | **Difficulty**: Easy

Nutrients per serving: Calories: 390 kcal | Fat: 33.79g | Carbohydrates: 5.47g | Protein: 17.66g | Fiber: 1.3g

Ingredients

8 oz cream cheese, softened (226 g)

2 tbsp minced cilantro

1/4 cup chopped green onion

1 lb chorizo (16 oz/ 453 g)

1 1/2 lb mushrooms (around 12 mushrooms) (24 oz/680g)

Method

1.   Preheat the oven to 350 °F.

2.   Cook and then cool the chorizo.

3.   Add the melted cream cheese, cilantro, and onions into a medium dish. With a slotted spoon, scrape the chilled chorizo

from the pan (leaving the oil behind) and add it to the dish's ingredients.

4.   Wash the mushroom caps and pat dry with the tea towel under hot water. By bending, remove the roots. (With a melon, widen the hole if necessary).

5.   Place the caps and stuff on a rimmed baking sheet with the mushrooms. To cover the crust, add plenty of water to the bottom and bake the mushrooms for about 20-30 minutes until they are browned.

6.   If you want additional browning, put it under the broiler. Remove carefully to the serving dish and serve sweet.

7.   With cling wrap, cover any remaining stuffed mushrooms and refrigerate. Microwave again or spray with foil and reheat for 20-30 minutes in a 350 F oven. Enjoy it within five days.

7 Graham Crackers With Almond Flour

Servings: 24 | **Time:** 27 mins | **Difficulty**: Easy

Nutrients per serving: Calories: 71 kcal | Fat: 6.4g | Carbohydrates: 2.6g | Fiber: 1.1g

Ingredients

2 1/2 Cups Almond Flour (250g)

1/2 cup + 2 Tbsp Monkfruit

2 1/2 tsp Baking powder

1/2 tsp Salt

1 Egg white

2 Tbsp Coconut oil, melted

2 tsp Molasses

Method

1.   Preheat the oven to 400 °F. Use parchment paper to cover a baking sheet. Stir together the monk fruit, baking powder, almond flour, and salt in a big cup. Add white, oil, and

the molasses to the egg and whisk until the sticky dough forms - it's best to blend with fingertips.

2.   On the table, place a large parchment paper's piece and put the dough on the top, covering it with another parchment paper's piece. Roll out to a thickness of just under 1/4 inch.

3.   Cut into 24 squares (approximately 3x3 inches) and put each square gently on the baking dish. Use a fork to softly stab the core on its own with a few holes.

4.   Bake for around 6-7 minutes until the sides are only golden brown (you will need to do them in 2 lots depending on your pan's size) but do not over-bake or get too hard when cold. Let the cool pan Full.

8   Cauliflower Pizza Crust

Servings: 2 | **Time:** 30 mins | **Difficulty:** Easy

Nutrients per serving: Calories: 342 kcal | Fat: 0.14g | Carbohydrates: 10.16g | Protein: 32.88g | Fiber: 3.6g

Ingredients

2 tbsp Whey Protein Powder (optional)

10 oz. of frozen cauliflower rice (thawed)

1/3 cup Kraft Parmesan cheese (in the can)

1-ounce cream cheese (28 g) (cut into small pieces)

1 large egg white

1 cup low moisture shredded mozzarella cheese (4 oz/ 113 g)
Optional Seasoning

1/4 tsp granulated garlic

1/4 tsp dried basil

1/4 tsp dried oregano

1/4 tsp fennel seeds

Method

1.   Preheat the oven to 425 °F. Place the rack in the middle. Line the parchment with a wide-rimmed baking sheet. Place the metal blade cutter in the food processor.

2.   Squeeze as much water as you can out of an empty bag of defrosted cauliflower rice on a clean, flat, tea towel. Up with your fingertips, fluff.

3.   Melt the mozzarella and cream cheese together for 1 minute in a healthy microwave dish. At 30- second intervals, stir and melt into molten. Now Scrape the cheese and add the white egg to the food processor. Process until smooth.

4.   Include and process the remaining ingredients before they fit together in a ball.

5.   Scrape up the cauliflower crust dough in the middle of a parchment-lined baking sheet with a rubber spatula.

6.   Pat, the dough in a 10-inch disc, ensuring that it is spread uniformly.

7.   Put in the oven the cauliflower pizza crust and bake for about 8-10 minutes or until one side is lightly browned. Flip over the crust and bake for 8-10 minutes. Control the crust closely so that the cheese does not burn.

8.   About 3-5 minutes or just until the cheese melts, cover the pizza with your desired toppings and transfer to the oven. Serve for your salad.

9 Chipotle Keto Deviled Eggs with Bacon

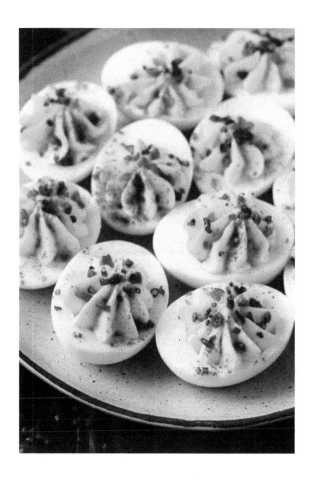

Servings: 12 | **Time:** 40 mins | **Difficulty:** Easy

Nutrients per serving: Calories: 26 kcal | Fat: 6.47g | Carbohydrates: 0.36g | Protein: 3.6g | Fiber: 0.1g

Ingredients

1 1/2 tbsp melted butter

1 tsp chipotle powder

1/2 tsp salt

1/4 tsp granulated garlic

2 tsp low carb powdered sugar (Swerve, Sukrin, Lakanto, Besti)
2 tsp sugar-free ketchup

3 tbsp mayonnaise

4 tsp white vinegar

6 large hard-boiled eggs

Topping:

2 tbsp minced cilantro

3 regular slices cooked bacon (crispy)

Paprika (for sprinkling)

Method

1.   Halve horizontally with the eggs. In a medium cup, scrape the yolks and place the half egg albumin on a platter or plate.

2.   With a fork, mash the yolks or drive them with the pan's backside into a fine sieve. Stir in the melted butter and the mayo, blending well.

3.   Apply the remainder of the ingredients to the filling and blend well to combine. Adapt the taste to your preference: lemon juice, sweetener to mellow and complement flavors, or salt to intensify flavors for more brightness. It is safest to let them stay overnight to blend the flavors. (You should cover the half egg whites at this stage and fill and refrigerate until appropriate the next day).

4.   Cover the halves with the egg and dust with paprika.

5.   Cut the bacon rather thinly, then drop it in a small dish. Mince up the coriander and weigh 2   tbsp. To remove some of the juice, put the cilantro in the folded paper towel, then squeeze it. It would not wilt or spill water in this manner.

6.   Mix the bacon, then cilantro, and scatter over each deviled egg uniformly. Cover and refrigerate softly or eat.

10   Shrimp Caprese Bites

Servings: 4 | **Time:** 10 days | **Difficulty**: Easy

Nutrients per serving: Calories: 79 kcal | Fat: 6g | Carbohydrates: 1g | Protein: 6g

Ingredients

1 1/3 ounce mozzarella cheese

1 tbs olive oil

1 tsp freshly squeezed lemon juice

12 basil leaves

12 extra-large cocktail shrimp

2 cherry tomatoes (cut into 8ths)

salt and pepper

Method

1.   in a small bowl, add shrimp mozzarella and whole cherry tomatoes. Add lemon juice and a tbsp of olive oil and season with pepper and salt to taste. To combine, toss.

2.   Cut the tomatoes into eighths and the balls of mozzarella into thirds.

3.   It would be best if you started assembling the skewers until the cheese and tomatoes are prepared. Insert a toothpick, right behind the tail, into the back of the shrimp. Then add a slice of tomato and mozzarella so that they stay in the shrimp's inner "c" shape. Fold up one leaf of basil and slip it on the toothpick. Finally, shift the toothpick to the other side of a shrimp.

4.   For each shrimp, repeat.

5.   Serve as is, or garnish with extra citrus, basil pesto, or the low carb vinaigrette instantly. Enjoy.

11   Low Carb Mozzarella Sticks

Servings: 4 | **Time:** 1 hr | **Difficulty:** Easy

Nutrients per serving: Calories: 94 kcal | Fat: 6g | Carbohydrates: 1g | Protein: 8g

Ingredients

1 egg beaten

1/2 tsp dried basil

1/4 tsp garlic powder

2/3 cup grated Parmesan cheese (the pasta aisle type)

8 sticks whole milk string cheese

Method

1.   Cut those sticks of cheese in two. Then smash the egg and lb it in a tiny bowl until it's all mixed. In another cup, weigh the Parmesan cheese. For the Parmesan cheese, add the basil and the garlic powder and whisk together to mix.

2.   First, dip the sliced mozzarella slice into a Parmesan mixture, then into the egg, and then into a Parmesan mixture again. On a baking sheet, put a dipped mozzarella stick on it.

Repeat unless you have dipped all the bits of mozzarella. For one hour, put the baking sheets in the fridge.

3. To 400 F, preheat the oven. For 8-10 minutes, bake the icy mozzarella sticks, turning once halfway. Serve hot, if desired, with tomato sauce. Enjoy

12 Pan Fired Turnips Recipe with Onions and Spinach

Servings: 4 | **Time:** 30 mins | **Difficulty:** Easy

Nutrients per serving: Calories: 84 kcal | Fat: 6.25g | Carbohydrates: 6.52g | Protein: 1.06g | Fiber: 2g

Ingredients

2 tbsp scallions

1/4 tsp salt

1/4 tsp pepper

1 tbsp olive oil

1 tbsp butter (or more olive oil)

1 sprig lemon thyme (or regular)

1 lb turnips

1 cup fresh spinach loosely packed

Method

1.   Peel and cut the turnips into quarters or sixths, if broad.

2.   Over medium fire, position a large frying pan. Apply the olive oil to a pan when heated and swirl it to coat. When the oil shimmers, add the turnips.

3.   Cook the turnips when one side is browned. Turn these over add to the pan with scallions and thyme. When the fork pierces, the thickest section slips quickly in the turnips.

4.   Apply the butter and spinach to the skillet and sauté before the spinach wilts. Has the thyme sprig removed?

5.   Season with pepper and salt, taste, and serve.

13   Bacon Wrapped Asparagus Bundles

Servings: 6 | **Time:** 31 mins | **Difficulty:** Easy

Nutrients per serving: Calories: 224 kcal | Fat: 46g | Carbohydrates: 7g | Protein: 21g | Fiber: 2g

Ingredients

olive oil spray

6 slices regular cut bacon

1 whole lemon, quartered

1 tsp lemon pepper

1 lb asparagus, trimmed (see post)

Method

1.   Preheat the oven to 400 °F. Put the rack in the center.

2.   If required, wash and dry the asparagus, peel, and trim. Split into 6 bundles.

3.   Wrap a slice of bacon in each package, slightly overlap the bacon, tuck the end under a bundle, and put it on a sheet tray. Using olive oil to spray and season with the lemon pepper.

4.   With the asparagus, put the quartered lemon on the sheet plate.

5.   Roast for eight minutes, turn over and roast for a full eight minutes. Crisp bacon under a broiler, if needed.

6.   Squeeze for service with a lemon.

14   Zucchini Pizza Bites

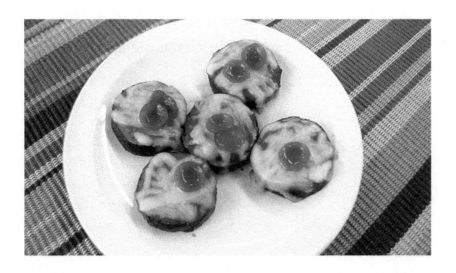

Servings: 12 mini pizzas | **Time:** 40 mins | **Difficulty:** Easy

Nutrients per serving (6 mini pizzas): Calories: 92 kcal | Fat: 7.2g | Carbohydrates: 3.6g | Protein: 4.4g | Fiber: 1.3g

Ingredients

1/4 cup Low Carb Marinara Sauce

1/4 cup Pitted Black Olives

1/2 medium Zucchini sliced into

12 rounds

1 slice Mozzarella Cheese or a vegan alternative like Daiya

Method

1.   To 350F, preheat the oven.

2.   In 12 1/4 inch slices, dice the zucchini. Place them on a tray for baking. Coat the slice with 1 tsp (or more/less per your preference) of marinara sauce.

3.   Cut an olive in half for making the spider pizzas for the body, then slice the other half into   the crescents to shape the legs. On the zucchini pizzas, arrange the olive bits.

4.   Assemble thin slices of the cheese and top the marinara to make mummy pizzas and put two olive slices.

5.   Bake now the pizzas for about 10 minutes or unless the cheese melts. Enjoy, enjoy.

15 Roasted Brussels Sprouts with Walnuts and Blue Cheese

Servings: 6 | **Time**: 40 mins | **Difficulty:** Easy

Nutrients per serving: Calories: 110 kcal | Fat: 8.25g | Carbohydrates: 6.93g | Protein: 4.35g | Fiber: 3g

Ingredients

1/4 tsp salt

1/4 tsp pepper

1/4 cup walnut pieces

1/4 cup crumbled blue cheese

1 1/2 tbsp olive oil divided use

1 lb Brussels sprouts (trimmed and quartered)

Method

1.   Preheat the oven to 400 °F. Shift the rack to the middle spot.

2.   Trim the Brussels sprouts and quarter them and position them in a medium dish. Mix the sprouts with 1 tbsp of olive oil, salt, and pepper.

3.   For 25-35 minutes, roast at 400°F, stirring half-way round. For the last 10 minutes, add the walnuts to the plate.

4.   Remove them from the oven and toss with the remaining oil in the serving bowl and change the seasoning.

5.   Just before serving, top with the crumbled blue cheese.

16   Keto Cornbread

Servings: 8 | **Time:** 40 mins | **Difficulty:** Easy

Nutrients per serving: Calories: 254 kcal | Fat: 20.4g | Carbohydrates: 5.2g | Protein: 13.7g | Fiber: 2g

Ingredients

3 large eggs (cold is fine)

2 cups almond flour (6.5 oz)

1/8 tsp salt

1/4 cup cream cheese, softened (2 oz)

1/2 tsp sweet corn extract

1 tbsp butter for the skillet

1 tbsp baking powder (or 1 1/2 tsp baking soda)

1 jalapeno

1 cup white cheddar cheese (or skim mozzarella) (4 oz)

Method

1.   Preheat the oven to 350°F. Put the rack in the center of the oven. Now Butter an 8-inch skillet of cast iron. (You will need an 8-inches baking dish, but it can differ in cooking time. Check for over-browning). Slice the jalapeno into dense circles of 1/8 inch.

2.   In a bowl of the food processor, put all ingredients for cornbread in order. Process the materials before a sticky dough emerges.

3.   Scrape the dough in a prepared skillet and scatter lightly over the sides and finish with slices of jalapeno.

4.   Bake for about 25-30 minutes or until gently browned at the tip. Until running a sharp and thin knife along the side and slicing to serve, remove it from the oven and cool for 10 minutes.

5.   Store the leftovers in the refrigerator in an air-tight bag. Reheat in a microwave or put on a baking sheet, then reheat a 300°F (about 15 minutes).

17 Keto Fried Green Tomatoes

Servings: 4 | **Time**: 35 mins | **Difficulty**: Easy

Nutrients per serving: Calories: 251 kcal | Fat: 19.5g | Carbohydrates: 3.2g | Protein: 13g | Fiber: 1g

Ingredients

3 tbsp olive oil (for frying)

2 large eggs, beaten

1 lb green tomatoes slices,

1/2-inch thick For dredging (optional)

1 tbsp whey protein powder (optional)

1 tbsp oat fiber (optional)

1/4 tsp pepper

1/4 tsp granulated garlic

1/4 tsp onion powder

1/2 cup grated Parmesan cheese (1 oz/ 29 g)

Keto Bread Crumb Coating:

1/2 tsp salt

1 cup crushed pork rinds (1 oz/ 29 grams) 1 tsp dried oregano

1 tsp dried basil

Method

1.   Place a slice on a wide sheet pan of waxed paper or parchment paper. Slice the tomatoes and let the paper towels drain on them.

2.   In a small dish, whisk together protein powder and the oat fiber (dredging blend, if using). Mix the ingredients for the keto bread crumbs and put them in a shallow dish. Beat the eggs with a fork in a shallow dish.

3.   With a fork, pick up the tomato slice and put it in a dredging mixture, covering both ends. Shake the waste off.

4.   Within the beaten egg, put these dredged tomato slices, covering both sides. Let drain off some waste.

5.   In the crumb mixture, put a wet tomato slice and cover both sides well. With crumbs, cover up the top side and press softly to ensure that they stick.

6.   Shift the tomato to the lined sheet pan, and the remaining slices of tomato remain to be sprayed.

7.   Over medium heat, heat a non-stick or a cast iron frying pan until clean. To coat the plate, apply 1 tbsp of oil and swirl. Add some tomato slices as the oil shimmers, then fry until browned. Switch the tomatoes, and the other hand is orange. As required, add more oil.

8.   To drain and cool when frying the remaining tomatoes, add the fried tomatoes to the paper towel or a cooling rack. Serve with a dipping sauce as a side or a dessert.

9.   Mix the mayo, siracha, powdered sweetener, and prepared horseradish (for a simple sauce to taste).

18 Baked Garlic Parmesan Chicken Wings

Servings: 4 | **Time:** 55 mins | **Difficulty:** Easy

Nutrients per serving: Calories: 512 kcal | Fat: 38.5g | Carbohydrates: 2.71g | Protein: 37.98g | Fiber: 0.75g

Ingredients

3 lb chicken wings, cut into pieces (about 11 whole wings)

1 cup grated Parmesan cheese (the good stuff - about 4 oz)

2 tbsp Garlic (or your favorite spice blend to taste)

1/2 cup mayonnaise

Method

1.   Cut each wing of the chicken into three parts: the wing, the drum, and the tip. Bone broth, discard all the tips, either pop in a bag and freeze.

2.   Preheat oven to 375 °F. Use foil or parchment paper to cover a wide sheet pan.

3.   In a medium shallow dish, mix 2 tsp of the seasoning mixture with the Parmesan cheese.

4.   Add mayonnaise to a big plastic zip bag, add bits of chicken wing, and seal. To uniformly coat each piece, maneuver the chicken wings with your hands. Instead, bring the mayo in a big bowl and cover the chicken with your mouth.

5.   Stab the wing with a fork and place it on seasoned Parmesan cheese. Coat a chicken wing with your hand and fork. On the lined sheet pan, put a chicken wing. Now repeat.

6.   Bake for about 40 minutes or until fully golden brown and baked through.

7.   If you use foil, quickly remove these chicken wings from the pan, or the cheese will adhere to the foil.

19 Oven-Fried Chicken Skin Cracklings

Servings: 4 | **Time:** 30 mins | **Difficulty**: Easy

Nutrients per serving: Calories: 126 kcal | Fat: 12g | Carbohydrates: 0g | Protein: 4.5g

Ingredients

8 raw chicken skin pieces from thighs or breasts

salt and pepper

seasoning of your choice

Method

1.   Remove the thighs or the chicken breasts from the chicken shell. With a knife, trim some big bits of fat off the sides. Underneath the skin, scrape away any additional fat or skin.

2.   Dry the skins thoroughly on paper towels and scatter in a single layer on the parchment paper.

3.   With the salt and pepper or your preferred spice, season gently. Go easy because the chicken's skin can shorten when it heats, focusing the seasoning (as much as 50 percent). In its fat, the chicken skin will fry.

4.   Bake for about 20 minutes or until the mixture is brown and crisp. Remove the extra fat from the pan and drain it on paper towels. Cool thoroughly and store in the fridge in an airtight jar. For several minutes, put on a sheet pan in the oven at 350 F to re-crisp if necessary.

20 Braised Escarole with Onions

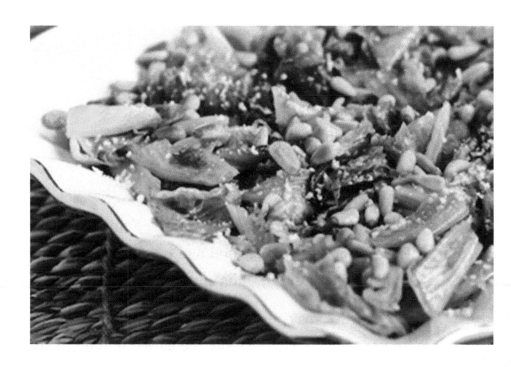

Servings: 4 | **Time:** 25 mins | **Difficulty:** Easy

Nutrients per serving: Calories: 124 kcal | Fat: 11g | Carbohydrates: 7g | Protein: 2g | Fiber: 4g

Ingredients

vinegar of your choice

Freshly ground black pepper

Diamond Crystal kosher salt

3 tbsp olive oil or ghee

1 onion thinly sliced

1 large head of escarole ~

2 lb 1 garlic clove minced

Method

1.   The first thing you have to do is isolate and wash the escarole leaves properly (lots of mud and dust can be there at the base of these inner leaves). Drain and cut coarsely.

2.   Heat the ghee over medium heat in a large skillet and sauté the onions until tender. Throw the garlic in and stir for about 30 seconds and then pour the escarole in it (damp greens are acceptable).

3.   The greens and the onions are finely salted and cooked until the leaves are wilted and soft (about 12-15 minutes). Add salt and pepper to season, and add a dash of your preferred vinegar.

21   Keto Cheese Chips

Servings: 6 | **Time**: 18 mins | **Difficulty:** Easy

Nutrients per serving: Calories: 74 kcal | Fat: 4.88g|
Carbohydrates: 0.61g | Protein: 6.76g

Ingredients

Herbs, spices, spice blends

4 oz Parmesan Cheese

Method

1.   Preheat the oven to 400 °F. Put the rack in the center
position. Line the parchment paper with   a large baking sheet.
If you don't have a grated Parmesan, process the cheese into fine
crumbles.

2.   Measure the tspful of cheese and put it on a parchment-
lined Panipat every mound of cheese softly (about 1 1/4 to 1 1/2
inches) in a circle with a finger. Until baking, dust with any
herbs, sauces, or flavorings.

3.   Cook the Parmesan crisps for 6 to 8 minutes before they
begin to turn golden brown. Let it cool fully for up to 30 days

before storing; put it in an airtight jar for about a week or in the fridge.

22   Rosemary Roasted Rutabaga

Servings: 4 | **Time:** 45 mins | **Difficulty:** Easy

Nutrients per serving: Calories: 100 kcal | Fat: 6.51g | Carbohydrates: 10g | Protein: 1.47g | Fiber: 3g

Ingredients

1 lb Rutabaga (peeled and cut into the 3/4-inch cubes)

1/8 tsp Freshly ground pepper

1/4 cup diced onion (1 oz)

1/4 tsp Salt

1 tbsp Chopped fresh rosemary

1 tbsp Olive oil

1 tbsp butter or ghee

Method

1.   Preheat the oven to 400 °F. Put the rack in the center. Using parchment paper to cover a sheet pan.

2.   Toss the onion, olive oil, pepper, rosemary, salt with the cubed rutabaga and spread it uniformly over the sheet pan. Bake about 20-30 minutes or until tender with a fork.

3.   Over lower heat, heat a medium to the large frying pan. Apply the butter and swirl when heated to coat the plate. Fry a rutabaga until browned lightly.

4.   To eliminate additional carbs, serve with fried, pan-seared, or roasted meat and a side salad.

23 Oven-Fried Parmesan Green Beans

Servings: 6 | **Time:** 30 mins | **Difficulty**: Easy

Nutrients per serving: Calories: 133 kcal | Fat: 9.88g | Carbohydrates: 6.19g | Protein: 5.3g | Fiber: 2.7g

Ingredients

Parmesan Green Beans

1/4 tsp salt

1/2 cup Parmesan cheese (Kraft in the can is fine)

1 lb green beans (stem end trimmed and dried with paper towels)

1 tsp minced garlic

1 large egg white (whipped until very frothy)

Sweet Mustard Dipping Sauce

1/4 cup mayonnaise (4 tbsp)

1/4 tsp dried dill, rubbed (or tarragon)

1/4 tsp pepper

1 1/2 tsp yellow mustard

1/2 tsp garlic salt

1/2 tsp smoked paprika (or regular)

2 tbsp sweetener of choice

Method

1.   Preheat the oven to 425 °F. Put the rack in the center spot. Using parchment paper to cover a large baking dish.

2.   In a shallow cup, mix these Parmesan cheese & minced garlic, and 1/4 tsp salt.

3.   In a large cup, put the green beans and toss with the white egg until fully coated. Add the combination of cheese and toss to cover.

4.   On the parchment-lined baking dish, scatter the green beans and sprinkle any leftover cheese on top.

5.   Bake around 15-20 minutes or unless the beans become cooked and browned with the cheese.

6.   Mix the ingredients for Sweet Mustard Sauce as the beans cook.

24   Crispy Pepperoni Chips

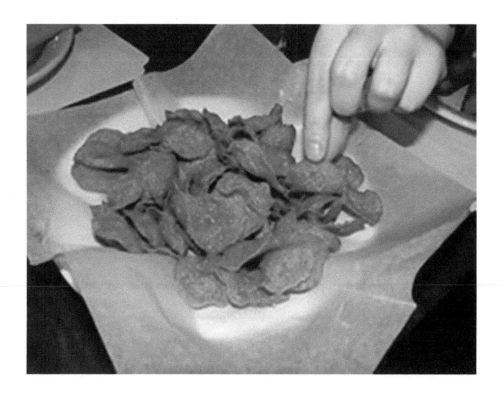

Servings: 1 | **Time:** 13 mins | **Difficulty:** Easy

Nutrients per serving: Calories: 150 kcal | Fat: 14g | Carbohydrates: 1g | Protein: 5g

Ingredients

15 Pre-sliced pepperoni slices (about one inch in diameter)

Method

Oven/Toaster Oven:

1.   Preheat the oven to 400 °F. 375 F for the toaster oven and place the rack in the center. Line parchment on a sheet pan. Put the pepperoni on a parchment, spread them evenly or if you're filling the sheet pan, let them just hit.

2.   Bake for 4 minutes. Be careful not to damage yourself with a paper towel—Bake for a further 4 minutes or until slightly browned with pepperoni. On a paper towel, remove and rinse.

Microwave:

1. Place the pepperoni on the paper towel on a healthy microwave plate and cook until crispy, at the interval of 20 seconds. Since microwaves differ in strength and wattage, the approximate time will rely on your microwave.

25   Tangy Ranch Chicken Wings

Servings: 4 | **Time:** 1 hr | **Difficulty**: Easy

Nutrients per serving: Calories: 341 kcal | Fat: 27.8g | Carbohydrates: 3g | Protein: 26g | Fiber: 2.4g

Ingredients

Olive oil spray

2 tsp olive oil

2 tsp Baking Powder

2 lb Chicken wing pieces

2 1/2 tsp Homemade Ranch Seasoning

1/4 tsp Salt

Method

1.   Preheat the oven to 375 °F with the middle rack in place.

2.   Dry the chicken wings with paper towels and place them in a wide dish.

3.   Mix 2 tsp of olive oil with the chicken wings once seasoned. Sprinkle the baking powder with 1 tsp and blend. Only repeat.

4.   Place the chicken wings over a wide sheet pan and skin-side-up on a wire rack. Bake the chicken for 40 minutes, flipping it halfway through.

5.   Take the chicken out of the oven and turn it upside-down again, for about 5-10 minutes just until the chicken is browned and crispy and put under the broiler.

6.   Take a big bowl of chicken and gently brush it with olive oil. Over the chicken, sprinkle 1 tsp of ranch seasoning and stir to cover. Repeat with the seasoning, but add 1/4 of a tsp of salt. Just serve.

26 Cabbage Noodles

Servings: 4 | **Time**: 20 mins | **Difficulty:** Easy

Nutrients per serving: Calories: 82 kcal | Fat: 5.9g | Carbohydrates: 7.3g | Protein: 1.8g | Fiber: 2.7g

Ingredients

1/4 cup onions, sliced thinly (1 oz)

1 lb cabbage (cored and cut into strips)

2 cloves garlic, sliced

2 tbsp butter or oil

salt and pepper to taste

Method

1.   Cut into quarters of the cabbage. Slice the onions thinly and peel the garlic.

2.   Over medium fire, heat a skillet. Apply the butter or oil when it is scorching and swirl to cover the plate. Add the cabbage, garlic, and onion and then saute until the cabbage becomes soft - about 10 minutes—salt to taste and pepper.

27 Oatmeal Sugar-Free Cookies

Servings: 20 | **Time**: 29 mins | **Difficulty**: Easy

Nutrients per serving: Calories: 119 kcal | Fat: 11.3g | Carbohydrates: 2.94g | Protein: 3.2g | Fiber: 1.8g

Ingredients

3/4 tsp cinnamon

1/4 tsp baking soda

1/4 tsp salt

1/3 cup Low carbohydrate brown sugar (50 g)

1/2 tsp of vanilla extract

1 1/2 cups sliced almonds (5 oz/142 g)

4 oz unsalted butter, softened (113 g)

1 cup of almond flour (95 g)

1 large egg, cold (room temperature)

2 tbsp of oat fiber (10 g)

2 tsp of grass-fed beef gelatin

Method

1.   Preheat the oven to 350 °F. Put the rack in the center position. Line parchment on a sheet pan. In a food processor or just by hand, cut sliced almonds to imitate the size of oats. Quantify and stir together the dry ingredients to remove the lumps.

2.   Sukrin Gold, vanilla extract, and Butter softened together until they become light and fluffy - around 1 1/2 minutes. Scrape the bowl down.

3.   At once, add all the dry ingredients and beat until mixed. Include the egg, and beat until mixed. The cut sliced almonds fold in.

4.   Scoop the dough and put on the baking sheet two inches apart using the 2 tbsp cookie scoop.

5.   Bake for 8 minutes, take from the oven, and softly bang a cookie sheet on the oven or counter to flatten the cookies - about 6 times. Keep in the oven for an extra 6 minutes.

6.   Take the cookies from the oven and use the spatula to slap each cookie gently. Before removing them from the cooling rack, let them cool for around 5 minutes. Until eating it, again cool these thoroughly.

28   Pulled Pork Stuffed Avocado Boats

Servings: 4 | **Time:** 15 mins | **Difficulty:** Easy

Nutrients per serving: Calories: 423 kcal | Fat: 34g | Carbohydrates: 9g | Protein: 23.5g | Fiber: 5g

Ingredients

1/4 cup BBQ sauce

1 1/2 cups pork or chicken (pulled)

2 avocados, halved and pitted

Garnish:

1 tbsp snipped chives or green onion

2 tbsp BBQ sauce (sugar -free)

2 tbsp ranch dressing (thinned slightly)

Method

1.   Halve the avocados and drain the pit. To make space for the filling, scoop out some of the avocados. (You may mash it

and blend it or put it on the top of pulled pork with a ranch dressing. I gave it to the children.)

2.   In a microwave or the frying pan, heat the pulled pork, and mix it with 1/4 cup of BBQ sauce of your choice. Dispense equally between the halves of the avocado.

3.   Drizzle each half with the remaining ranch dressing and BBQ sauce. Add chives or green onion to garnish.

4.   You can eat as it is or pop put it in the microwave to warm it. Alternatively, put in a 350 F preheated oven and bake for around 20 minutes, sealed. Cover some leftovers and refrigerate them.

29 Sweet Bell Pepper Salad

Servings: 6 | **Time:** 15 mins | **Difficulty:** Easy

Nutrients per serving: Calories: 112 kcal | Fat: 9g | Carbohydrates: 6.4g | Protein: 2g | Fiber: 2g

Ingredients

2 oz feta cheese crumbled

2 oz. onion, sliced thinly

1/2 tsp garlic, minced

1 lb mixed bell peppers, sliced

1 fennel bulb, sliced thinly

Dressing:

1 pinch pepper

1/2 tsp Fines Herbs (basil, tarragon, parsley, dill)

1/4 tsp salt

2 tbsp Champagne vinegar (you can also use rice wine vinegar)

3 tbsp extra virgin olive oil

Method

1.　　Cut and soak each onion in 1/4 cup of water and 2 tbsp of white vinegar for 10-15 minutes if you use heavy onions. Drain, use, again.

2.　　Cut the vegetables into a medium-large serving bowl and add them.

3.　　Mix up the dressing ingredients. Ensure that the fines herbs are rubbed on your palm or rubbed on your fingers to crack the flavor to extract it.

4.　　To change the seasoning, toss, and taste. Apply the cheese to the feta and toss gently. Only serve it cold.

30 Keto Baba Ganoush

Servings: 8 | **Time:** 55 mins | **Difficulty:** Easy

Nutrients per serving: Calories: 81 kcal | Fat: 6g | Carbohydrates: 6.3g | Protein: 2.3g | Fiber: 3.3g

Ingredients

1/4 cup Greek yogurt

1 large eggplant, sliced lengthwise (1 1/2 lb)

2 tsp minced garlic (1-2 cloves)

1/2 tsp ground cumin

2 tbsp tahini paste

2 tbsp extra virgin olive oil

1 tbsp lemon juice

salt and pepper to taste

Method

1.   Preheat the oven to 400°F. Please put it in the middle spot on the oven rack. Using parchment paper to cover a sheet pan.

2.   Lengthwise, slice the eggplant, salt generously, and leave to rest for 15 minutes to remove the bitter juices. Quickly scrub, then pat dry. When pierced with a fork, put the eggplant having cut side down, then roast for 45 minutes or when the eggplant is fully tender. Remove and cool from the oven

3.   Scoop the skin from the soft eggplant pulp and put it in a food processor. Now Pulse to split-up. Include the other ingredients and process until the dip becomes smooth and creamy in the blender.

4.   Taste the seasoning and adjust. Serve right away, or cover and refrigerate for up to five days. The next day it tastes better. Serve mildly warm like room temperature.

31   Low Carb Keto Taco Shells

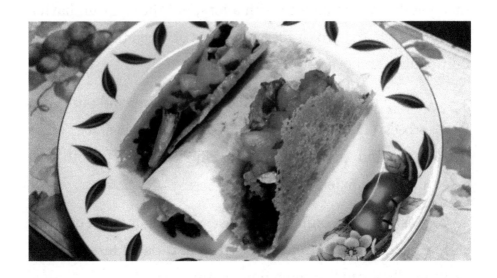

Servings: 6 | **Time:** 25 mins | **Difficulty:** Easy

Nutrients per serving: Calories: 171 kcal | Fat: 13.6g | Carbohydrates: 1g | Protein: 10.6g

Ingredients

9 oz pre-shredded cheddar cheese

Method

1.   Put one rack in the upper third and the other rack in the lower third of the oven and preheat the oven to 375 °F. Using parchment paper to cover two wide sheet pans. (Flip the parchment over so that the cheese doesn't have a pencil or pen.)

2.   Quantify 1/3 cup (1 1/2 ounce) per circle of shredded cheese and spread uniformly over the sides of the circle.

3.   Bake about 5 minutes and swap the baking sheets' places. Bake for another 5-10 minutes, or until the cheese layer has small holes and the edges tend to tan.

4.   Before removing onto wooden spoons or the spatulas supported by glasses to form taco shells, remove from oven and blot with the paper towel. Leave for chalupa or the tostada shells to cool flat on the pans.

5.   Cool thoroughly and place for a few days in an air-tight jar. Or for up to two weeks in the refrigerator.

32 Low Carb Peanut Butter Balls

Servings: 20 | **Time:** 10 mins | **Difficulty**: Easy

Nutrients per serving: Calories: 104 kcal | Fat: 6g | Carbohydrates: 2g | Protein: 8g | Fiber: 1g

Ingredients

1 1/3 cup whey protein powder

1/2 tsp stevia glycerite

1 cup smooth peanut butter

Method

1.   In a medium cup, add the ingredients and blend (knead) with the rubber spatula until thoroughly mixed.

2.   Pinch-off sized sections of the dough with walnut and roll into the balls.

3.   Up to 10 days in an airtight jar placed in the refrigerator.

33 Mexican Green Beans

Servings: 6 | **Time**: 25 mins | **Difficulty:** Easy

Nutrients per serving: Calories: 84 kcal | Fat: 7g | Carbohydrates: 6g | Protein: 1g | Fiber: 3g

Ingredients

1/4 cup chopped onion (1 oz)

1 tsp fresh oregano, minced (or 1/4 tsp of dry but fresh tastes different)

1/4 tsp ground cumin

1/2 cup Roma tomato, seeded and diced (4 oz)

1 lb green beans, trimmed and cut

1 clove garlic, minced

2 tbsp avocado oil or good olive oil

1 tbsp butter, ghee, or another tbsp of oil

2 tbsp water

1 whole bay leaf, crumbled

1 tsp chicken base

salt and pepper to taste

Method

1.   Wash the beans, strip them, and cut them. To separate seeds, split the tomato in half, squeeze carefully over the garbage, and then dice. Chop the onion, ginger, mince, and fresh oregano (if using).

2.   Heat 1 tbsp of oil over medium heat in a large frying pan. Add the onion, tomato, garlic, and bay leaf when it is hot until the onion starts to soften. Add water, oil, oregano, green beans, and cumin, and for another tbsp to the chicken's base. Whisk to coat the beans and use a sheet of foil or a cap to cover them loosely. Cook for about 4 minutes or when the beans become cooked or according to your preference.

3.   Apply butter, add garlic, pepper, or more oregano and the cumin to change the seasoning. Now serve.

34 Broccoli Fritters With Cheddar Cheese

Servings: 4 | **Time:** 18 mins | **Difficulty:** Easy

Nutrients per serving: Calories: 204 kcal | Fat: 16g | Carbohydrates: 5.8g | Protein: 12g | Fiber: 3g

Ingredients

1 cup shredded cheddar cheese

1 Tbsp avocado oil

1 tsp Cajun seasoning

2 large eggs, beaten

2 Tbsp oat fiber or almond flour, or the powdered pork rinds

8 oz. broccoli (cut into small pieces or chopped)

Method

1.   Cut the crowns of fresh broccoli and stems into half-inch by half-inch sections. In the oven or a steamer, steam gently. If damp, remove any extra water and then dry with paper towels. (Drain well and cut into small bite-sized bits if surplus broccoli is used.)

2.   With the flour of your choosing and a Cajun seasoning, toss or swirl the broccoli to coat. Mix the egg and stir. Apply the cheddar cheese and whisk until mixed thoroughly.

3.   Once heated, put a cast iron or the non-stick pan on medium heat. To oil the pan, apply the oil, and swirl. Less oil is essential for a non-stick pan. The mixture is visually separated into fourths and spooned into the tray, placed in a low mound or a patty. Back into the piles, scrape some tumbled pieces.

4.   In one hand, cook until the cheese starts to melt on top of the patty and the bottom becomes crusty brown around 2-3 minutes. Flip and sear until browned on the other hand.

5.   Serve with an egg or a dipping sauce on top.

35 Low Carb Hamburger Buns

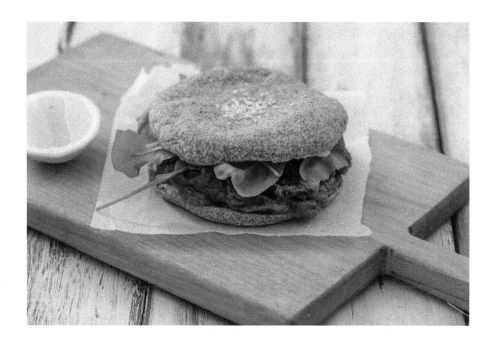

Servings: 5 | **Time:** 23 mins | **Difficulty**: Easy

Nutrients per serving: Calories: 294 kcal | Fat: 25g | Carbohydrates: 7g | Protein: 14g | Fiber: 3g

Ingredients

2 tbsp oat fiber (or protein powder or 1/4 c. more almond flour)

2 oz cream cheese

1 tbsp baking powder

1 large egg

1 1/4 cup almond flour

1 1/2 cup part-skim grated mozzarella cheese

Method

1.   Place the cream cheese and mozzarella cheese in a healthy microwave bowl, then microwave   for about 1 minute. Whisk and microwave for an extra 30 seconds to 1 min. Scrape the cheese along with the egg into a food processor and process until they become smooth.

2.   Include the dry ingredients, then process them until they form a dough. It's pretty sticky. Let it cool for a few minutes if it's too hot to touch.

3.   Preheat the oven to 400 °F. Put the rack in the center of the oven. Cover a sheet with parchment for baking. At the bottom of an oven, put a cheap metal pan.

4.   Cut into 5 sections equal to each other. Lightly oil your hands and roll each piece into a ball. Place your hand on the parchment paper and softly flatten it slightly while still maintaining the domed shape.

5.   At the bottom of an oven, put 6 ice cubes in a metal tray. Then the rolls are put in the oven.   That will help raise and disperse the rolls.

6.   Bake for about 12 minutes or until golden brown on the outside. These will be soft still, so before removing them from the baking sheet, let them cool. Store in the refrigerator after cooling. Slightly warm for pleasure.

7.   Hold the burger buns in an air-tight jar in the refrigerator. They can be stored for 7-10 days and freeze well too.

36 Crispy Fried Eggplant Rounds With Parmesan Cheese and Marinara Sauce

Servings: 4 | **Time:** 30 mins | **Difficulty:** Easy

Nutrients per serving: Calories: 233 kcal | Fat: 17.26g | Carbohydrates: 7.15g | Protein: 11.38g | Fiber: 4g

Ingredients

1 cup crushed pork rinds (1 oz/ 28.35 g)

1 lb eggplant (cut crosswise into 1 cm - 1/2 inch rounds, 453.6 g)
1 tsp dried basil

1 tsp dried oregano

1/2 cup grated Parmesan cheese (1 oz/ 28.35 g)

1/2 tsp salt

1/4 tsp granulated garlic

1/4 tsp onion powder

2 tbsp olive oil

2 large eggs, beaten

1/4 tsp pepper

Method

1.   Preparation: Put the eggplant in 10-12 rounds, sprinkle with salt, and leave to drain for 15 minutes in a colander. Dry full-on towels with paper. Meanwhile, in a shallow bowl (soup or cereal bowl), put the eggs wide enough to hold an eggplant round and scramble with the fork. In another small dish, blend the pork rinds, cheese, and seasoning. Get a little sheet pan packed.

2.   Procedure: Use a fork to pick up around and flip this back and forth along the egg until fully coated. Grab a fork and let the egg fly away. Place in the crumb mixture, and crumbs cover the end. To the end, click the crumbs. Then use the fork to turn the round over and do this again. Raise the round eggplant and shake the excess crumbs. Lay yourself on a pan of paper. On all of the rounds, repeat the process. Depending on how large they are, you should've enough for 10-12 rounds.

3.   Cook: Over medium-high cook, heat an iron skillet or non-stick pan. Alternatively, a large pancake skillet may be used, and both fit on the skillet at once. Add the oil when it is hot (you will need much less oil in a non-stick skillet). When the oil becomes hot, add 3-4 rounds to the pan and cook on either side for 3 minutes. To rinse, switch to a paper towel and then to a cooling rack. You may have to add a few more oil to the skillet as you go or adjust the heat just slightly. It'll be brown and crispy

with the eggplant. Serve with hot mayo, tomato sauce, or serve as it is.

37 Easy Low Carb Roll

Servings: 8 | **Time:** 18 mins | **Difficulty**: Easy

Nutrients per serving: Calories: 165 kcal | Fat: 13g | Carbohydrates: 3g | Protein: 10g | Fiber: 1g

Ingredients

2 tbsp whey protein powder (or oat fiber or coconut flour or 1/4 cup more almond flour)

2 oz. cream cheese, cubed

1 tsp baking soda (or 1 tbsp of baking powder)

1 large egg

1 1/4 cup almond flour

1 1/2 cup shredded skim mozzarella cheese

Method

1.   a microwave-safe dish, melt the cream cheese and mozzarella together for 1 minute at maximum strength. Stir, then heat for a further 30-45 seconds to melt. Scrape the cheese into a food processor's bowl and process until mixed completely. Add the egg and whisk until mixed.

2.   The food processor adds the dry ingredients and process until thoroughly mixed (about 10-15 seconds).

3.   Using oil to spray a sheet of cling film to scrape the bread dough into the middle of the cling film. It's VERY STICKY. Shape the dough softly into a disc or oval and cool it in the freezer until the oven is ready. (NOTE: the dough doesn't have to go into the freezer if it's not sticky.)

4.   Preheat an oven to 400 °F. Put the rack in the center of the oven. Line a piece of parchment or Silpat with a baking sheet.

5.   Remove the dough from the freezer when the oven is ready, and cut it into 8 pieces. The dough would stick to the knife-like crazy. It's all right.

6.   To flatten the rim, softly oiled your hands, carefully roll the dough portion into a ball and lower it onto the prepared cookie sheet. For the remaining dough, reverse the procedure. Sprinkle with sesame, poppy, or dehydrated onion seeds, pressing very softly to bind to the dough.

7.   Bake for 13-15 minutes, roughly. It will brown the dough, and it will break. Enjoy, enjoy. Hold the extra rolls in the fridge (or freezer) and warm them gently before feeding.

38   Asparagus with Hollandaise Sauce

Servings: 4 | **Time**: 15 mins | **Difficulty**: Easy

Nutrients per serving: Calories: 248 kcal | Fat: 26g | Carbohydrates: 3g | Protein: 4g | Fiber: 1g

Ingredients

salt and pepper to taste

1 tbsp water

1 lb asparagus, trimmed Hollandaise Sauce

1 tbsp water

1/2 tsp Dijon mustard

1-2 pinch cayenne pepper

1-2 pinch white pepper

1-2 tsp freshly squeezed lemon juice (or white vinegar)

2 large egg yolks

4 oz. salted butter

Method

1.   If the asparagus' thickness is medium-large, cut 1 inch from the bottom and use a vegetable peeler to gently peel the

stalks. Start from the top at around 1/3 and proceed at the bottom of every spear. Keep a spear at the bottom. If the asparagus is thin, then bend it until it snaps. Split to the same length as the remaining bows. Separate the eggs for another use, reserving the whites.

2.   In a microwave-safe dish, put the asparagus and add 1 tbsp of water. Cover with the plastic wrap and cook, depending on the microwave, at high power for 1 1/2 - 2 1/2 minutes. Drain the water out to leave it hidden. Alternatively, in boiling broth, blanch the asparagus until crisply tender, rinse, and keep warm.

3.   In a mixer, mix the egg yolks, 1 tbsp of water, 1 tsp of lemon juice, and mustard. Put the lid on top, then remove the piece from the center. In a medium-sized to the large frying pan, put the butter and melt the butter over a medium flame. Turn the heat to medium-high and rotate the pan softly every couple of moments. Turn the heat off as the solids at the bottom of a pan start to turn brown. Turn the blender down and start pouring that hot butter in the blender, leaving behind the brown solids in the pan.

4.   Add the white pepper and cayenne pepper after the butter has been absorbed, and mix. With more vinegar, salt, or pepper, change the seasoning. Pour on the asparagus and quickly eat.

39   Green Beans Almondine

Servings: 4 | **Time**: 15 mins | **Difficulty:** Easy

Nutrients per serving: Calories: 177 kcal | Fat: 16g | Carbohydrates: 9g | Protein: 3g | Fiber: 4g

Ingredients

salt and pepper to taste

4 tbsp butter

1/4 cup flaked or slivered almonds

1 tbsp lemon juice

1 lb trimmed green beans Optional (any, not both)

1 clove garlic, minced

1 tbsp shallots, minced

Method

1.   Preparation: Wash & trim the green beans for a good appearance, cutting on the bias. Mince when using garlic or the shallots. To make squeezing simpler, roll a lemon on the table.

2.   Beans: Put the green beans with 1-2 tbsp of water in the microwave-safe dish and cover with a clinging wrap. Microwave until practically crisp-tender for 2-3 minutes; the duration will depend on the microwave. Drain and stir the water. To release gas, leave it exposed.

3.   Boil a pot of water and keep a big bowl of ice water standing by the Conventional method. Add the green beans while the water is boiling and cook when crisp-tender and light green. To stop frying, pour the beans and drop them directly into the ice bath. Drain them a little and dry them.

4.   Over medium heat, put a large saute pan and add the almonds and butter. Cook just until the almonds have just started to brown. (Add now and mix until fragrant if using garlic cloves or shallot). Add the green beans immediately and stir in the butter to cover. All the way through, steam the beans, then squeeze lemon juice over them. To taste and serve, add salt and pepper.

40 Spicy Jalapeno Coleslaw

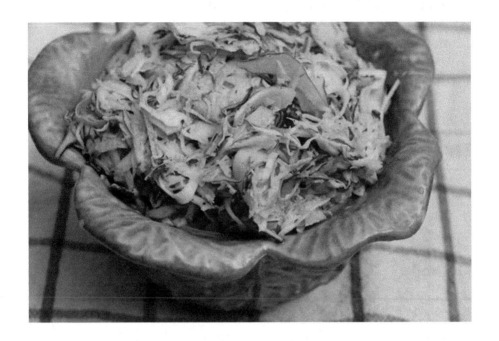

Servings: 10 | **Time**: 15 mins | **Difficulty**: Easy

Nutrients per serving: Calories: 109 kcal | Fat: 10g | Carbohydrates: 4g | Protein: 1g | Fiber: 1g

Ingredients

¼ cup Mayonnaise

¼ cup Red Bell Pepper, julienned

¼ cup Yellow Bell Pepper, julienned

½ tsp Chili powder

1 Jalapeno pepper, seeded and finely diced

1 lime, juiced

1 tbsp Cilantro, minced

1/2 cup Ranch dressing

2 oz. Red cabbage, finely sliced

8.5 oz. Coleslaw mix

Method

1. Toss the coleslaw mixture, red bell pepper, jalapeno pepper, and yellow bell pepper together in a big dish.

2. Mix the ranch dressing, lime juice, mayonnaise, chili powder, and cilantro in a shallow dish.

3. Using the slaw to spill the dressing over and toss to cover.

4. Until serving, refrigerate for about 30 minutes.

41   Cucumber Avocado Tomato Salad

Servings: 10 | **Time:** 15 mins | **Difficulty:** Easy

Nutrients per serving: Calories: 136 kcal | Fat: 12g | Carbohydrates: 8g | Protein: 2g | Fiber: 4g

Ingredients

¼ cup Olive Oil

¼ cup Red Wine Vinegar

½ Red Onion

½ tsp Salt, plus more to taste

1/4 tsp Black pepper,

2 Avocados

2 large Cucumber

3 tbsp Lime juice

4 large Tomatoes

Method

1.   Cut the vegetables into bite-size pieces.

2.   In a little mug, mix the olive oil, vinegar, salt, lime juice, and pepper.

3.   In a wide dish, toss the cucumbers and tomatoes together and then spray the seasoning over them, turning them until all is well seasoned.

4.   Add the bits of avocado and fold them carefully into the salad.

5.   Immediately serve.

42   Easy Pickled Cauliflower

Servings: 8 | **Time:** 2 days 20 mins | **Difficulty:** Easy

Nutrients per serving: Calories: 39 kcal | Fat: 1g | Carbohydrates: 6g | Protein: 1g | Fiber: 1g

Ingredients

1 small Cauliflower

1 cup White vinegar

1 cup Apple cider vinegar

2 cups Water

4 cloves Garlic

2 Tbsp Sugar, (or sugar substitute)

1 tbsp Kosher salt

2 tbsp Mustard seed

2 tsp Coriander seeds

1/2 Red Pepper

1/2 orange bell pepper

¼ tsp Red pepper flakes

2 tsp Black peppercorns

Method

1.   Divide a sliced cauliflower into 2 wide mouths pint mason jars and bell peppers equally.

2.   In a small pot, add vinegar, water, garlic, sugar, coriander, mustard seeds, peppercorns, salt, and red pepper flakes and put to a boil on medium-high heat.

3.   Remove it from heat until the mixture hits a boil and let it cool about 5 minutes before pouring it into each jar. Make sure that in each container, you have an equal distribution of spices.

4.   Before screwing a lid on and sticking the jars in the fridge, let that mixture cool completely. Let it rest for 24 to 48 hours before eating.

43   Italian Antipasto Skewers

Servings: 12 | **Time:** 10 mins | **Difficulty**: Easy

Nutrients per serving: Calories: 224 kcal | Fat: 46g | Carbohydrates: 7g | Protein: 21g | Fiber: 2g

Ingredients

8 oz. Primo Taglio Mozzarella Cheese

5 oz. Artichoke Hearts

3 oz.Primo Taglio Prosciutto

24 leaves Fresh Basil

2 oz. Primo Taglio Italian Sliced Salame (Dry)

16 oz.Roasted Red Peppers

12 Olives

Method

1.   Split three strips of 1/2 inch mozzarella. Cut the slices into 4 quarters each.

2.   Cut 6 lengthwise artichoke hearts in half.

3. On a 5 inch skewer, arrange the ingredients. Start with a slice of salami. To form a wedge shape, fold it in half and then again in half. Push on the skewer for that.

4. thA slice of folded basil accompanies it, then a wedge of mozzarella cheese as well as the other folded basil leaf.

5. Now Cut roasted red pepper into the 1-inch wide strip 2-inch high, fold and slip onto the skewer.

6. Roll it up and cut a piece of prosciutto in two. Press it on the skewer, preceded by half of the artichoke's heart and one of the olives.

44   Oven Roasted Cabbage Steaks

Servings: 6 | **Time:** 40 mins | **Difficulty**: Easy

Nutrients per serving: Calories: 125 kcal | Fat: 10g | Carbohydrates: 9g | Protein: 3g | Fiber: 4g

Ingredients

1/4 cup Olive oil

1 head Cabbage

2 tbsp Parmesan (finely grated)

1 clove Garlic (finely minced)

½ tsp Crushed red pepper flakes

½ tsp Kosher Salt

Method

1.   Cut cabbage into half-inch-thick slices, then put it on a baking sheet lined with foil.

2.   Mix the olive oil, parmesan cheese, garlic cracked red pepper flakes, and salt together in a shallow cup.

3.   Slightly covering each side, brush the mixture on the cabbage slices.

4.   Bake for 15 minutes in an oven at 400°F. Flip the slices of cabbage and finish baking for a full 15 minutes.

45 Keto Colcannon

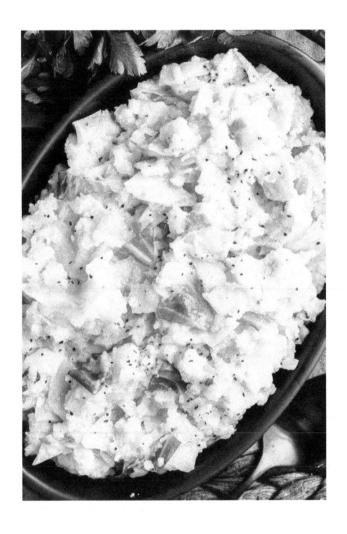

Servings: 12 | **Time:** 15 mins | **Difficulty**: Easy

Nutrients per serving: Calories: 58 kcal | Fat: 4g | Carbohydrates: 5g | Protein: 2g | Fiber: 2g

Ingredients

Salt to taste

6 oz. cabbage (cut into thin 1-inch long slices)

4 tbsp butter, divided

36 oz. Cauliflower, chopped

Method

1.   To a simmer, put a big pot of water. Add the cauliflower and let it simmer for 10 minutes or so. You will feel that when it is soft to quickly split off with a fork, the cauliflower is finished.

2.   Melt 1 tbsp of butter in the large skillet while the cauliflower is cooking. Include the cabbage and saute until softened for 5-7 minutes.

3.   When the cauliflower has done frying, pour the water into a strainer and rinse it thoroughly. To eliminate water as possible, let it stay for several minutes.

4.   In the empty cup, pour a cauliflower back in and add cabbage and the leftover butter. Marinate together until the consistency of mashed potato.

5.   To taste, apply salt and serve.

46 Keto Blueberry Scones

Servings: 8 | **Time:** 33 mins | **Difficulty:** Easy

Nutrients per serving: Calories: 110 kcal | Fat: 8g | Carbohydrates: 6g | Protein: 2g | Fiber: 2g

Ingredients

3/4 cup Almond flour

1/4 cup Coconut flour

1/4 tsp salt

1/4 cup butter, unsalted, softened

1/4 cup Almond Milk (Unsweetened)

5 tbsp Granular erythritol sweetener

2 tsp gluten-free baking powder

2 tsp Vanilla extract

1 large Egg

1 cup Blueberries

Method

1.   Preheat the oven to 350 °F.

2.   Mix all the dry ingredients in the bowl of your blender (except the chocolate chips).

3.   Include the softened butter and milk it until it is well combined and there are no bits of butter along with the dry ingredients.

4.   Include the vanilla extract, almond milk, and egg and begin combining until well mixed.

5.   Apply the blueberries and then roll them into the dough using a spatula.

6.   Shape 2.5 oz of dough into a triangle shape with your palm. Place a cookie sheet on an unoiled one. Repeat until you consume all of the dough. Approximately 8 scones you can receive.

7.   Bake for 18-23 minutes or when the sides are golden brown in the oven at 350 °F. You start to see some golden brown patches on top.

8.   Takeout from the oven and leave to fully cool the scones before placing them in an airtight jar.

47   Cheesy Bacon Brussels Sprouts

Servings: 6 | **Time**: 35 mins | **Difficulty**: Easy

Nutrients per serving: Calories: 261 kcal | Fat: 23g | Carbohydrates: 8g | Protein: 8g | Fiber: 3g

Ingredients

6 slices cooked bacon, chopped

4 tbsp Olive oil

2 oz. Cheddar cheese

1.25 tsp salt, divided

1 lb Brussels sprouts

½ tsp Onion powder

½ tsp Garlic powder

½ cup Heavy cream

¼ tsp Salt

Method

1.   Preheat the oven to 375° F.

2.   Over medium heat, heat a large size oven-safe skillet.

3.   Add the olive oil and the sprouts from Brussels. Sprinkle with 1 tsp of salt and simmer until the sprouts appear to soften and brown in patches, for about 10 minutes.

4.   Mix the heavy cream, garlic powder, onion powder, and the remaining 1/4 tsp of salt as the brussels sprouts become cooked.

5.   Remove them from the sun until the Brussels sprouts are prepared and pour a heavy cream mixture on them.

6.   Sprinkle the Brussels sprouts with cheddar cheese and bacon over them.

7.   Place the skillet in an oven until the cheese is fully melted and bake for 10 minutes.

48 Keto Chocolate Chip Scones

Servings: 8 | **Time:** 30 mins | **Difficulty:** Easy

Nutrients per serving: Calories: 156 kcal | Fat: 20g | Carbohydrates: 5g | Protein: 2g | Fiber: 2g

Ingredients

4.5 oz. Lily's Dark Chocolate Chips

3/4 cup Almond flour

1/4 cup Coconut flour

1/4 tsp salt

1/4 cup butter, unsalted, softened

1/4 cup Unsweetened Almond Milk

5 tbsp Granular erythritol sweetener

2 tsp gluten-free baking powder

2 tsp Vanilla extract

1 large Egg

Method

1.   Preheat the oven to 350 °F.

2.   Mix all of the dry ingredients in the bowl of your blender (except for the chocolate chips).

3.   Apply the softened butter and milk it until it is well combined, and there are no bits of butter along with the dry ingredients.

4.   Apply the vanilla extract, almond milk, and egg and begin combining until well mixed.

5.   Include the chocolate chips and then roll them into the dough using a spatula.

6.   Shape 2.5 oz of dough into a triangle shape with your palm. Place a cookie sheet on an unoiled one. Repeat until you consume all of the dough. Approximately 8 scones you can receive.

7.   Bake for 17-21 minutes or until the sides are golden brown in the 350 °F ovens, and you have to see golden brown patches on top. Remove from the oven and leave to fully cool the scones before placing them in an airtight jar.

49 Classic Cheese Ball Recipe

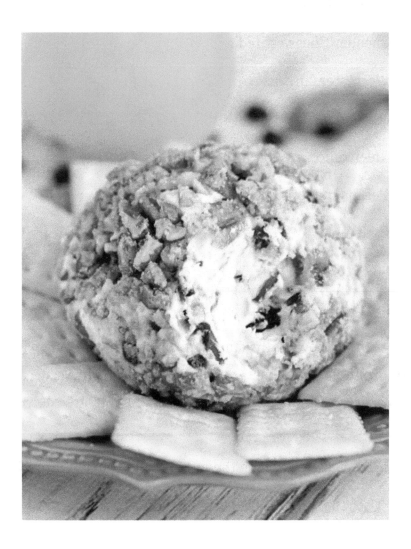

Servings: 10 | **Time:** 10 mins | **Difficulty**: Easy

Nutrients per serving: Calories: 238 kcal | Fat: 22g | Carbohydrates: 3g | Protein: 8g | Fiber: 1g

Ingredients

8 oz. Cream Cheese, softened

8 oz. Cheddar Cheese shredded

2 tsp Worcestershire sauce

1 tsp Lemon juice

1 tsp Green onion, finely chopped

1 cup Pecans, roughly chopped

¼ tsp Salt

Method

1.   1.In the bowl of the stand mixer, put the cream cheese, green onion, cheddar cheese, Worcestershire sauce, salt, lemon juice, and blend until all the ingredients are thoroughly mixed.

2.   Scrape the bowl with the mixture and shape it into a ball.

3.   Use the chopped pecans to roll the ball until it is completely enclosed.

4.   Cover the ball of cheese in plastic wrap and put for 1 hour in the refrigerator to cool.

5.   Serve with crackers and vegetables.

50 Air Fryer Chicken Wings

Servings: 4 | **Time:** 40 mins | **Difficulty:** Easy

Nutrients per serving: Calories: 375 kcal | Fat: 31g | Carbohydrates: 1g | Protein: 23g | Fiber: 1g

Ingredients

1 tsp Pepper

1/2 cup Frank's Red Hot Sauce

1/4 cup butter, melted

2 lb Chicken wings (cut into drumettes and flat)

2 tsp salt

Method

1.   Pat's chicken drumettes and the wings dry with a paper towel and put them on the baking sheet or a cutting board.

2.   Sprinkle salt and pepper on the chicken.

3.   Put the chicken in an air-fryer basket and cook for 25 minutes at 380 °F. Cut the basket halfway through and use

tongs to dip the chicken around and shift it around so that bottom reaches the top.

4.   Turn the heat to 400 °F after 25 minutes and continue cooking for 5 minutes or when the skin is crispy.

5.   Take the chicken from the basket and put it in a wide bowl with the fryer.

6.   Over the chicken wings, add the sauce and throw them until well seasoned.

7.   Immediately serve.

Lightning Source UK Ltd.
Milton Keynes UK
UKHW021359070521
383304UK00001B/48